Dyslexia for Kids

Complete Users Manual in Bringing Out the Best

in Dyslexic Kids and Adults (Brain Imaging)

Julie D. Hall

Table of Contents

INTRODUCTION

Regardless of the many confusions and misunderstandings, the word dyslexia is often utilized by medical personnel, researchers, and clinicians. Among the most typical misunderstandings concerning this condition is that dyslexia is an issue of attention, or term reversals (b/d, was/noticed) or of characters, words, or sentences "dance around" on the web page (Rayner, Foorman, Perfetti, Pesetsky, & Seidenberg, 2001).

Dyslexia can be an often-misunderstood, confusing term for reading problems. The term dyslexia comprises of two different parts: **dys-** *abnormal, or impaired* or *difficult*, and **-lexia** signifying *words, reading, or vocabulary*. So quite actually, ***dyslexia*** means difficulty with words (Catts & Kamhi, 2005).

Actually, writing and reading words backwards are normal in the first stages of understanding how to read and write among average and dyslexic children as well, and the existence of reversals may or might not indicate an underlying reading problem.

Probably one of the most complete definitions of dyslexia originates from over twenty years of research:

- Dyslexia is a particular learning impairment that is neurobiological in the source. It is seen as a problem with accurate and/or fluent phrase acknowledgement, and poor spelling and decoding capabilities. These troubles typically derive from a deficit in the phonological element of vocabulary that is often unpredicted with regards to other cognitive skills and the provision of effective classroom training. (Lyon, Shaywitz, & Shaywitz, 2003)

- Dyslexia is a particular learning impairment in reading that often impacts spelling as well. Actually, reading impairment is the most common and most carefully analysed study of the training disabilities, influencing 80% (eighty percent) of most specified learning disabilities. As a result of this, we use the conditions: *dyslexia and reading disabilities* (RD) interchangeably in this specific article to spell it out to the students.

It really is neurobiological in origins, and therefore the problem is situated physically in the mind. Dyslexia is not triggered by poverty, developmental hold off, conversation, hearing impairments, or learning another vocabulary, although those conditions may put a kid more in danger of creating a reading impairment (Snow, Burns, & Griffin, 1998).

Children with dyslexia will most likely show two apparent problems when asked to learn text message at their quality level. First, they'll not have the ability to read much of the text message; you will see many words which they'll stumble, think of, or try to "audio out." This is actually the problem with *"fluent term recognition"* identified in the last definition.

Second, they will show decoding difficulties, and therefore their attempts to recognize words they don't know will produce many mistakes. They'll not be very accurate in using letter-sound associations in mixture with context to recognize unknown words.

These problems in phrase recognition are credited to a

fundamental deficit in the sound element of language, that means it is very hard for readers connecting characters and sounds to be able to decode. People who have dyslexia frequently have trouble comprehending what they read because of the fantastic difficulty they experience in accessing the imprinted words.

Common Misunderstandings about Students with Reading Disabilities

1. Writing words backwards are symptoms of dyslexia.

2. Writing characters and words backwards are normal in the first stages of understanding how to read and write among average and dyslexic children. It is an indicator that orthographic representations (i.e. forms and spellings of words) have never been firmly founded, and a child with this characteristic commonly has reading impairment (Adams, 1990).

Reading disabilities are triggered by visual belief problems.

The existing consensus predicated on a big body of research (e.g., Lyon et al., 2003; Morris et al., 1998; Rayner et al., 2001; Wagner & Torgesen, 1987) is that dyslexia is most beneficially characterized as a problem with vocabulary digesting at the phoneme level, with no problem with visual digesting.

In the event that you just provide them with plenty of time, children will outgrow dyslexia.

There is absolutely no evidence that dyslexia is a problem that may be outgrown. There is certainly, however, strong proof that children with reading problems show an ongoing prolonged deficit in their reading, rather than simply developing later like average children (Francis, Shaywitz, Stuebing, Shaywitz, & Fletcher, 1996). More strong proof demonstrates that children with dyslexia continue steadily to experience reading problems into adolescence and adulthood (Shaywitz et al., 1999, 2003).

More males than ladies have dyslexia.

Longitudinal research implies that as much girls as boys are influenced by dyslexia (Shaywitz, Shaywitz, Fletcher,

& Escobar, 1990). There are numerous possible known reasons for the over identification of men by colleges, including higher behavioural performance and a smaller capability to play among kids. More research is required to determine why.

Dyslexia only impacts people who speak British.

Dyslexia appears in every cultures and dialects in the world with written vocabulary, including the ones that do not use an alphabetic script such as Korean and Hebrew. In British, the principal difficulty is accurate decoding of unfamiliar words. In constant orthographies such as German or Italian, dyslexia shows up more regularly as a problem with fluent reading - people may be accurate, but very decrease (Ziegler & Goswami, 2005).

People who have dyslexia will reap the benefits of coloured text message overlays or lens.

There is absolutely no strong research evidence that mentioned using coloured overlays or special lens has any influence on the term reading or comprehension of children with dyslexia (American Optometric

Association, 2004; Iovino, Fletcher, Breitmeyer, & Foorman, 1998).

A person with dyslexia can't ever figure out how to read.

This is not true. The sooner children who struggle are recognized and provided organized, intense teaching, the less severe their problems will tend to be (Country wide Institute of Child Health insurance and Human Being Development, 2000; Torgesen, 2002). With properly intensive instructions, however, even teenagers with dyslexia may become accurate, albeit decrease people (Torgesen et al., 2001).

What regions of the mind relate with language and reading?

The mind is a complex organ that has many different functions. It sets the body and receives, analyses, and stores information.

The brain can be divided down the centre lengthwise into the right and a left hemisphere. A lot of the areas accountable for talk, language digesting, and reading are in the left hemisphere, and because of this we will concentrate our explanations and numbers on the still left side of the brain. Within each hemisphere, we find the next four brain lobes.

The frontal lobe is the biggest and accountable for controlling speech, reasoning, planning, regulating emotions, and consciousness.

In the 19th century, Paul Broca was discovering areas of the mind used for language and observed a particular area of the brain that was impaired in a guy whose speech became limited after a stroke. This area received increasingly more attention, now we realize that Broca's area, located within the frontal lobe, is very important to the organization, creation, and manipulation of vocabulary and conversation (Joseph, Noble, & Eden, 2001). Regions of the frontal lobe are also very important to silent reading skills (Shaywitz et al., 2002).

The parietal lobe is situated farther behind the brain and controls sensory perceptions as well as linking spoken and written language to memory to provide it meaning so we can know very well what we hear and read.

The occipital lobe, at the trunk of the head, is where in fact the primary visual cortex is situated. Among other styles of visual understanding, the visible cortex is important in the recognition of letters.

The temporal lobe is situated in the lower area of the brain, parallel with the ears, and it is involved with verbal memory.

Wernicke's area, long regarded as important in understanding vocabulary (Joseph et al., 2001), is situated here. This region, determined by Carl Wernicke at a comparable time and using the same methods as Broca, is crucial in language digesting and reading.

Furthermore, converging evidence shows that two other systems, which process vocabulary within and between lobes, are essential for reading.

The foremost is the left *parieto-temporal* system that are involved with word analysis - the conscious, effortful decoding of words (Shaywitz et al., 2002). This region is crucial along the way of mapping words and written words onto their audio correspondences - notice noises and spoken words (Heim & Keil, 2004). This area is also very important to comprehending written and spoken vocabulary (Joseph et al., 2001).

The next system that is very important to reading is the still left *occipito-temporal* area. This technique appears to be involved in automated, rapid usage of whole words and it is a crucial area for skilled, fluent reading (Shaywitz et al., 2002, 2004).

Exactly what does brain imaging research reveal about dyslexia?

<u>Structural brain differences</u>

Studies of structural variations in the brains of individuals of all age groups show distinctions between people who have and without reading disabilities.

The brain is chiefly composed of two types: ***grey matter and white matter***. *Grey matter* is exactly what we see whenever we take a look at a brain and is mainly made up of nerve cells. Its main function is digesting information.

White matter is available within the deeper elements of the mind, and comprises of connective fibres protected in myelin, the coating made to facilitate communication between nerves. *White matter* is mainly accountable for information transfer in the brain.

Booth and Burman (2001) found that individuals with dyslexia have less grey matter in the left parieto-temporal area than non-dyslexic individuals. Having less grey matter in this area of the brain may lead to problems digesting the sound framework of vocabulary (phonological consciousness).

Many people who have dyslexia likewise have less white matter in this same area than average readers, which is important because more white matter is correlated with an increase of reading skill (Deutsch, Dougherty, Bammer, Siok, Gabrieli, & Wandell, 2005). Having less white matter could lessen the power or efficiency of the parts of the brain to talk to one another.

Other structural analyses of the brains of individuals with and without RD have found variations in hemispherical asymmetry. Specifically, most brains of right-handed, non-dyslexic people are asymmetrical with the still left hemisphere being bigger than the same area on the right.

On the other hand, Heim and Keil (2004) discovered that right-handed people who have dyslexia show a pattern of symmetry (right equals left) or asymmetry in the other direction (right bigger than left). The precise reason behind these size variations is the main topic of ongoing research, however they appear to be implicated in the reading and spelling problems of individuals with dyslexia.

CHAPTER 1

Fast Facts on Dyslexia

Individuals who have dyslexia frequently have a problem finding out how to read and write.

· Dyslexia isn't linked to cleverness.

· Early diagnosis, guidance, and support can lessen the impact of dyslexia.

· People who've dyslexia will establish immunological problems.

What's Dyslexia?

Dyslexia commonly causes complications in word reputation, spelling, and decoding.

Inside a person with dyslexia, the mind processes written materials differently. This can make it exist hard to recognize, spell, and decode words.

Individuals who have dyslexia have problems

understanding what they read. Dyslexia is a neurological and sometimes genetic condition, as opposed to the result of poor teaching, training, or upbringing.

Between five and fifteen percent of people in the us have dyslexia.

Diagnosis

If a father or mother, guardian, or instructor suspects a youngster may have dyslexia, they need to ask in the child's college with regards to a professional evaluation. Early analysis is a lot much more likely to result in effective treatment.

Test results may possibly also open the entrance way to more support for a child; they could become qualified to get special education services, support programs, and services in universities and colleges.

Diagnostic tests often cover another areas:

· background information.

· Intelligence.

·   dental language skills.

·   word recognition.

·   decoding, or the ability to read new words through the use of letter-sound knowledge.

·   phonological processing.

·   automaticity and fluency skills.

·   reading comprehension.

·   vocabulary knowledge.

·   genealogy and early development

Through the assessment process, the examiner will need to have the capability to eliminate other conditions or conditions that may show similar symptoms. For example eyesight problems, hearing impairment, insufficient instruction, sociable and financial factors.

Symptoms

Dyslexia differs from delayed reading development

which can reflect mental impairment, or cultural deprivation.

The most typical indicators connected with dyslexia could be displayed at any age, nonetheless they normally occur within childhood.

Child years' symptoms of dyslexia include:

·   Difficulty in finding out how to read

Many children with dyslexia have normal intelligence and receive proper teaching and parental support, nonetheless they have difficulty finding out how to read.

·   Milestones reached later

Children with dyslexia may work out how to crawl, walk, chat, and trip a bike later than almost all others.

·   Delayed speech development

A youngster with dyslexia usually takes much longer period to determine how exactly to speak, and they also may mispronounce words, find rhyming challenging, and appearance to never distinguish between different term sounds.

- Decrease at learning units of data

At college, children with dyslexia usually takes longer time to understand the characters from the alphabet and just how they might be pronounced. There may be problems keeping in brain the changing times from the week, weeks of 4 seasons, colours, and several arithmetic tables.

- Coordination

The kid can happen clumsier than their peers. Obtaining a ball could be difficult. Poorer eye-hand coordination could be considered an indicator of additional similar neurological conditions, including dyspraxia.

CHAPTER 2

Symptoms of Dyslexia

Indicators of dyslexia could be difficult to recognize before your kid enters school, however, many early clues may indicate a problem. Once your kid reaches school age, your kid's teacher could be the first to see a problem. Severity varies, however, the problem often becomes apparent as a youngster starts finding out how to read.

Before School

Signs a young child may be susceptible to dyslexia include:

- Late talking

- Learning new words slowly.

- Problems forming words correctly, such as for example reversing sound in words or confusing words that sound alike.

·   Problems remembering or naming words, digits and colours.

·   Difficulty learning nursery rhymes or getting involved in rhyming games.

School Age

Once your kid is within college, dyslexia indicators could be more apparent, including:

·   Reading well below the expected level for age.

·   Problems controling and understanding what they hear.

·   Difficulty discovering the proper phrase or forming answers to questions.

·   Problems remembering the group of things.

·   Difficulty viewing (and occasionally hearing) similarities and variations in characters and words.

·   Inability to voice out the pronunciation of a fresh word.

·   Difficulty spelling.

·   Spending an unusually long time completing tasks that involve reading or writing.

·   Staying from actions that involve reading

Teenagers and Adults.

Dyslexia symptoms in teenagers and adults become those in children. Some common dyslexia indicators in teenagers and adults include:

·   Difficulty reading, including reading aloud.

·   Sluggish and labour-intensive reading and writing

·   Problems spelling.

·   Staying away from actions that involve reading

·   Mispronouncing titles or words, or problems retrieving words.

·   Trouble understanding jokes or expressions that have a meaning not easily comprehended from the complete words (idioms).

·   Spending an unusually long time completing tasks that involve reading or writing.

·   Difficulty summarizing an account.

·   Trouble learning a Spanish.

·   Difficulty memorizing.

·   Difficulty doing mathematics problems

When to see a doctor

Though most children decide to learn reading at kindergarten or 1st grade, children with dyslexia often can't grasp the basics of reading by that time. Talk with a medical doctor if your kid's reading level is below what's expected in relation to generation, or in the event that you see additional signals of dyslexia.

When dyslexia goes undiagnosed and untreated, child's many years of reading difficulties continue into Adulthood.

Risk Factors of Dyslexia

Dyslexia risk factors include:

·   A family background of dyslexia or other learning disabilities.

·   Premature delivery or low delivery weight.

·   Exposure during carrying a child to smoking, drugs, alcohol consumption or contamination that may alter brain development in the foetus.

·   Person distinctions in the components of the mind that allow reading

·   Complications.

Dyslexia can lead to plenty of problems, including:

·   Trouble learning: Because reading can be an art basic to numerous various other school topics, a youngster with dyslexia reaches a disadvantage for most classes and may possess trouble maintaining peers.

·   Social problems: Left untreated, dyslexia can result in low self-esteem, behavioural problems, stress, aggression, and drawback from friends, parents and instructors.

·   Problems as adults: The shortcoming to understand and comprehend can prevent a youngster from reaching his/her potential as a child grows up. This might own long-term educational, interpersonal and economic outcomes.

·   Children who've dyslexia are in increased risk of having attention-deficit/hyperactivity disorder (ADHD), and vice versa. ADHD could cause difficulty sustaining attention as well as hyperactivity and impulsive behavior, which can make dyslexia harder to deal with.

CHAPTER 3

What Can Cause Dyslexia?

Dyslexia is not actually an illness; it's a problem from delivery, and it often happens in families. Individuals who have dyslexia aren't ridiculous or sluggish. Most have average or above-average cleverness, and they also work very difficult to conquer their learning problems.

Research demonstrates dyslexia is because of the type of brain information. Pictures of the mind display that whenever individuals who have dyslexia read, they use various regions of the mind than people without dyslexia. These pictures also demonstrate that this brains of people with dyslexia don't work effectively during reading. In order that is the reason why reading seems like such sluggish effort.

How are you affected in Dyslexia?

Most people think that dyslexia causes visitors to change letters and figures and read words backwards. But reversals happen as a typical part of development, and also have emerged in lots of kids until first or second stage.

The principal problem in dyslexia is trouble recognizing phonemes. They will be the basic sound of conversation (the "b" audio in "bat" is a phoneme), so that it is challenging to make the connection in the middle of your audio and see symbol for the sound, and to blend sound into words.

This helps it be hard to recognize short, familiar words or to sound out longer words. It needs lots of period for any person with dyslexia to audio out a term because term reading takes more time and concentration. A person with dyslexia is often lost during term reading, and reading understanding is poor.

It is not surprising that folks with dyslexia have trouble spelling. Furthermore, they may possess trouble expressing themselves in writing as well as speaking. Dyslexia is a vocabulary processing disorder, so that it is important in every types of vocabulary: spoken or written.

A lot of people have milder types of dyslexia, so they could have less trouble in the regions of spoken and written vocabulary. A lot of people work around their dyslexia, nonetheless it requires a lot of effort and additional work. Dyslexia isn't a thing that goes away completely or a person just outgrows. Luckily, with proper help, a lot of people who have dyslexia work out how to read. They often times find other ways to understand and make use of those strategies their lives.

What it is to have Dyslexia?

When you yourself have dyslexia, you've got trouble reading even simple words you've seen often. You most likely will read gradually and think that you must work extra hard when reading. You might mix in the letters in a nutshell - for instance, reading the word "now" as "received" or "left" as "experienced". Words may possibly also blend collectively and areas are lost.

You've got trouble remembering what you've read. You may remember easier when the same information is read for you personally or you hear it. Phrase problems in mathematics could be especially hard, even though you have mastered the basics of arithmetic.

If you're performing a demonstration prior to the class, you've got trouble discovering the proper words or names for various objects. Spelling and writing tend to be extremely hard for folks with dyslexia.

How is Dyslexia Diagnosed?

Individuals who have dyslexia often get methods to work around using their impairment, so nobody will know they're having difficulty. This may save some embarrassment, but obtaining help can make school and reading easier. Many folks are diagnosed as kids, nonetheless it isn't unusual for teens and even adults to become diagnosed.

A teen's parents or educators might suspect dyslexia if indeed they notice several problems:

· poor reading skills, despite having normal intelligence.

·   poor spelling and writing skills.

·   trouble finishing projects and checks within time limits.

·   difficulty remembering the proper brands for things.

·   trouble memorizing written lists and telephone numbers.

·   issues with directions (informing from quit or up from down) or reading maps.

·   trouble getting through Spanish classes

Having among the problems doesn't imply you have dyslexia. But someone who shows several indications ought to be examined for the problem.

A physical exam, including hearing and eyesight tests, will be performed to remove any medical problems. A college psychologist or learning specialist should give several standardized tests to measure language, reading, spelling, and writing abilities. Sometimes a test of thinking ability (IQ test) is given. A lot of people with dyslexia own trouble in other school skills, like handwriting and math, or they could have trouble attending to or remembering things; if this can be a case, other styles of testing may be achieved.

How exactly to Cope with Dyslexia

Although coping with dyslexia could be difficult, help is available. Under authorities law, someone informed they have a learning impairment like dyslexia is qualified to receive extra support from everyone in the school system. A youngster or teen with dyslexia usually must start using a specially trained teacher, tutor, or reading specialist to comprehend how exactly to learn and spell better.

The best sort of help teaches knowing of speech sounds in words (called phonemic awareness) and letter-sound correspondences (called phonics). The instructor or teacher should use special learning and practice activities for dyslexia.

Students with dyslexia gets more time to complete projects or tests, permission to record class lectures, or copies of lecture notes. Employing a computer with spelling checkers certainly are a good notion for written assignments. For older students in challenging classes, services could be by offering recorded versions of any book, even textbooks. Applications that "reads" printed material aloud can be obtainable, ask your parent, teacher, or learning disability services coordinator methods for getting these services if you'd like them.

Emotional support is essential. Individuals who have dyslexia often get frustrated because regardless of how hard they try, they can not appear to maintain with other students. They could think that they're significantly less wise as their peers, and may cover their problems by performing up in course or being the course clown. They will make an attempt to get additional students to accomplish their work to them. They could pretend that they don't really actually value their grades or that they think school is dumb.

Family and friends can help individuals who have dyslexia by realizing that they aren't stupid or lazy, plus they should try as hard because they can. It is advisable to identify and appreciate each person's talents, whether they're in athletics, drama, art, creative problem solving, or one more thing.

Individuals who have dyslexia shouldn't look small within their academics or career choices. Most colleges make special accommodations for students with dyslexia, offering them trained tutors, learning aids, applications, recorded reading assignments, and special arrangements for exams. Individuals who have dyslexia could become doctors, politicians, corporate executives, actors, musicians, artists, teachers, inventors, entrepreneurs, or other activities that they select. Many celebrities with dyslexia have very successful careers in these and other fields, despite having had reading struggles in school.

CHAPTER 4

Can Dyslexia be cured?

In a nutshell, No. Dyslexia is a lifelong condition that impacts people into old age. However, that will not imply that education cannot remediate some of the affected individuals who have dyslexia with written vocabulary. A large body of proof shows what types of training struggling readers need to be successful (e.g., Country wide Institute of Child Medical health insurance and Person Development, 2000; Snow et al., 1998; Torgesen, 2000).

Now analysts may also "appearance" in the brains of children before and after a rigorous intervention and discover for the first time the consequences from the intervention on the mind activity of children with RD.

Listed here are two of such studies.

Aylward et al. (2003) imaged ten children with dyslexia and eleven average people before and after a twenty-eight-hour treatment that only the students with dyslexia received. They likened both sets of students on out-of-magnet reading assessments aswell as the quantity of activation during duties of identifying notice sounds.

They found that as the control children showed no distinctions between two imaging, the students who received the task showed a considerable increase in activation, in the areas very vital that reading and language through the phonological task. Before the intervention, the youngsters with RD demonstrated significant under-activation in these areas in comparison to the control children, and following a treatment, their profiles were virtually identical.

These results should be viewed with caution due to many limitations. One limitation is usually having less specificity about the participation that was provided, another may be the tiny test size, as well as the last is having less an experimental control group (i.e., many children with RD who didn't possess the procedure). Lacking any experimental control group, we can not ensure that the procedure triggered the changes within the mind activation due to so many other possible explanations.

Shaywitz et al. (2004) resolved these restrictions within their analysis of brain activation changes before and after an involvement. They examined seventy-eight second and third graders with reading disabilities who was simply randomly designated to three organizations:

- the experimental intervention.

- school-based remedial programs.

- Control.

CHAPTER 5

20 Common Dyslexia Symptoms

Children can begin showing indicators of the learning impairment when in preschool years. While every case of dyslexia is exclusive to the average indivdual, you'll find so many common characteristics and behaviours from the dyslexic. We've put together a listing of twenty of the very most typical dyslexia symptoms to assist you identify if your kid reaches risk level.

Remember that several are symptoms of dyslexia, not causes of dyslexia. They may be outlined in no particular order.

- Problems with reading.

- Difficulty spelling words in writing products.

- Low Self-confidence or behavioural problems.

- Letter and/or quantity reversals (transposing).

- Issues with pronunciation.

- Omitting sound or words when reading and writing.

- Issues of headaches.

- Difficulty reading aloud.

- Confusion left and right.

- Issues with writing tools like pencils or pens.

- Trouble with sequenced instructions.

- Guessing, missing or updating words instead of sounding out.

- Strong dental comprehension and poor reading comprehension.

- Letters on a page could possibly move, appear "blurry" or "out of place".

- Difficulty with business and time management.

- Failure to differentiate talk sounds.

- Difficulty repeating phrases or sentences.

- Humiliated by grades.

- Flash bank cards and memorization don't work.

- Reading below quality level or peers

CHAPTER 6

Strengths of Dyslexia

Seeing the larger picture

Individuals who have dyslexia often see things more holistically. They miss the trees but begin to start to see the forest.

"It's as if individuals who have dyslexia tend to make use of a wide-angle contact lens to consider the world, while some tend to utilize a telephoto; each is usually most appropriate at uncovering various kinds of fine details". Matthew H. Schneps, Harvard University

Locating the unusual one out

Individuals who have dyslexia master global visual handling as well as the recognition of impossible statistics. Dyslexic scientist Christopher Tonkin explained his unusual degree of sensitivity to "things out of place". Researchers in his kind of work must sound right of enormous degrees of visible data and accurately find dark hole anomalies.

There are increasing numbers of people with dyslexia in neuro-scientific astrophysics. It prompted research in the Harvard-Smithsonian Centre for Astrophysics. Results verified that people which have dyslexia are better at determining and memorizing complicated images.

Improved pattern recognition

Individuals who have dyslexia can handle observing how things attach to create organic systems, and to identify similarities among multiple things. Such advantages will have a tendency to exist of particular significance for areas like technology and mathematics, where visible representations are key.

"I recognized I had formed dyslexia, and I promptly realized I had developed this present for imaging. I have a home in a world of patterns and images, and I see things that nobody else sees. Because of dyslexia, I possibly could discover these patterns."

"You can't overcome it (dyslexia); you can work around

it and make it work for yourself, nonetheless it never goes away completely. That's probably an essential thing, because if dyslexia travelled away, in that case your additional presents would disappear completely too."

Sound spatial knowledge

Many individuals who have dyslexia demonstrate better skills at manipulating 3D objects within their mind. Many of the world's top architects and fashion designers have dyslexia.

Advantages to Dyslexia

"I have been called stupid. Not only can i not read, but I couldn't memorize my assignment work. I used to be always in underneath from the class. I became very depressed." Richard Rogers

"We performed poorly at college - once I attended, I had been regarded to as stupid due to my dyslexia. I nonetheless possess trouble reading. I have to concentrate very difficult at going quit to ideal, left to right; normally my vision just wanders within the website." Tommy

Hilfiger

Picture Thinkers

Individuals who have dyslexia tend to think in pictures instead of words. Research on the University of California has proven children with dyslexia have improved picture recognition storage.

Nineteenth-century French sculptor, Auguste Rodin, could stare at paintings in museums by day, and paint them from storage at night time. His dyslexia designed he could not read or write by age fourteen, together with his reading skills developing much later.

Sharper peripheral vision

Individuals who have dyslexia have better peripheral eyesight than most, meaning they are able to easily ingest an entire scene. Though it could be hard to focus in on specific words, dyslexia may actually make it better to find external edges.

Business entrepreneurs

Do you realize one in three American companies have dyslexia?

Companies like Thomas Edison, Henry Ford, Steve Jobs and Charles Schwab were all dyslexic. Perhaps better strategic and creative considering could provide an actual business benefit.

"I seemed to think in various ways from my classmates. I have been very centered on trying to make a company and create something. My dyslexia led precisely how we communicated with customers." Richard Branson

Highly Creative

Many of the world's most creative stars have dyslexia, such as for example Johnny Depp, Keira Knighltly and Orlando Bloom.

"Many of the super developers I've met appeared to employ an essential aspect in keeping their experience from dyslexia." Soren Petersen, Design Research Ph.D.

Pablo Picasso (Designer)

Picasso was described by his educators as "having difficulty differentiating the orientation of characters". Picasso colored his topics as he noticed them - sometimes out of order, backwards or ugly. His paintings verified the power of his creativity, that was perhaps from the shortcoming to find out written words properly.

Thinking away from package - problem solving

Some people that have dyslexia are popular for having unexpected leaps of insight that solve problems with an unorthodox approach.

That's an intuitive approach to problem solving that may look like daydreaming. Looking from your windows is how dyslexics work, allowing their brain put on natural and simplicity around a problem to let contacts assemble.

CHAPTER 7

What's Brain Imaging?

Several techniques are available to visualize brain anatomy and function. A trusted tool is magnetic resonance imaging (MRI), which creates images that may reveal information regarding brain anatomy (e.g., the amount of grey and white matter, the integrity of white matter), brain metabolites (chemicals within the mind for communication between brain cells), and brain function (where large pools of neurons are energetic). Functional MRI (fMRI) would depend around the physiological theory that works in the mind (where neurons are "firing")k connected with a growth of blood flow in comparison to that specific section of the brain. The MRI sign bears indirect information regarding raises in blood flow. Out of this transmission, researchers infer the positioning and amount of activity that's associated with a task, such as for example reading solitary words, that the analysis participants are undertaking in the scanner.

Data from these studies are often collected on groupings of people instead of individuals for research purposes, only-not to diagnose people who have dyslexia.

Which Brain areas get worked up about Reading?

Since reading is a cultural invention that arose following an evolution of modern humans, no location within the mind acts as a reading center. Instead, brain locations that sub serve other functions, such as for example spoken vocabulary and object identification, are redirected (instead of innately given) for the purpose of reading (Dehaene & Cohen, 2007). Reading entails multiple cognitive procedures, two which were of particular interest to analysts:

1) grapheme-phoneme mapping where mixtures of characters (graphemes) are mapped onto their related sound (phonemes) and that are thus "decoded".

2) visible word form acknowledgement for mapping of familiar words onto their mental representations. Collectively, these methods allow us to pronounce words

and access meaning. In accordance with these cognitive procedures, studies in adults and children have exhibited that reading is backed having a network of areas in the quit hemisphere, just like the occipito-temporal, temporo-parietal, and substandard frontal cortices. The occipito-temporal cortex keeps the "visible phrase form area". Both temporo-parietal and poor frontal cortices tend to involve with phonological and semantic digesting of words, with poor frontal cortex also confusing in formation of talk sound. These areas have already been which can change after generation (Turkeltaub, et al., 2003) and so are modified in individuals who have dyslexia (Richlan et al., 2011).

What have brain images revealed about brain framework in dyslexia?

Evidence of a connection between dyslexia as well as the framework of the mind was initially discovered by examining the anatomy of brains of deceased adults who had dyslexia throughout their lifetimes. The left-greater-than-right asymmetry typically seen in the left hemisphere temporal lobe (planum temporale) was not within these brains (Galaburda & Kemper, 1979), and ectopias (a displacement of brain cells to the very best of brain) were mentioned (Galaburda, et al., 1985). Then researchers began to use MRI to discover structural images in the brains of research volunteers with and without dyslexia. Current imaging techniques have exposed less grey and white matter quantity and changed white matter integrity in quit hemisphere occipito-temporal and temporo-parietal areas. Experts remain looking at how these email address details are influenced using a person's vocabulary and writing systems.

What have brain images revealed about brain function in dyslexia?

Early functional studies were tied to adults because they employed invasive techniques that are looking into radioactive materials. The field of brain mapping greatly benefited from invention of fMRI. fMRI won't require the use of radioactive tracers for this to become safe for children and adults, and may be used frequently which facilitates longitudinal studies of development and involvement. First used to examine dyslexia in 1996 (Eden et al., 1996), fMRI offers since been trusted to examine the brain's role in reading and its particular components (phonology, orthography, and semantics). Studies from different countries have converged in results of modified left-hemisphere areas (Richlan et al., 2011), including ventral occipito-temporal, temporo-parietal, and second-rate frontal cortices (and their contacts). Results from the studies confirm the universality of dyslexia across different world dialects.

Think about genes, brain chemistry, and brain function?

Many hereditary variants are connected with dyslexia, and their influence on the brain continues to be investigated in people and mice. Using pets which were bred to have genes connected with dyslexia, experts went into how these genes might impact development of and communication among brain location. These investigations dove-tail with studies in humans.

Variations in brain anatomy (Darki, et al., 2012; Meda et al., 2008) and brain function (Deal et al., 2012; Pinel et al., 2012) have already been seen in individuals who bring dyslexia-associated genes, actually those people who have sound reading skills. Furthermore, to these investigations in the anatomical, physiological, and molecular amounts, research workers need to pinpoint the substance link with dyslexia. For example, brain metabolites that tend to be involved with allowing neurons to communicate could be visualized using another MRI-based technique called spectroscopy. Several metabolites (for instance, choline) are often different in individuals who have dyslexia (Pugh et al., 2014). Experts continue to explore the connections between these results and so are hopeful that what they learn will determine the resources of dyslexia. That is clearly a difficult element of research because distinctions in the brains of people with dyslexia aren't always the reason behind their reading issues (for instance, it could also certainly be a consequence of reading less).

Adjustments in Reading, Changes in the mind

Brain imaging research has revealed anatomical and functional changes in typically developing people because they work out how to read (e.g. Turkeltaub et al., 2003); additionally it is revealed in children and adults with dyslexia pursuing effective reading education (Krafnick, et al., 2011; Eden et al., 2004). Such studies also shed light onto the brain-based variations of children with dyslexia who reap the advantages of reading instruction compared to those who don't produce benefits. Neuroimaging data are also used to forecast long-term reading success for children with and without dyslexia.

Causes vs Consequences

A key point of research on the mind and reading is to see whether the findings would be the cause or the consequence of dyslexia. Many of the brain areas associated with dyslexia will also be changed by finding out how to read, as shown by evaluations of adults who've been illiterate but discovered to understand

(Carreiras et al., 2009). Longitudinal studies in typical people uncover anatomical changes with generation, a few of that are linked to development (Giedd et al., 1999) as well as others towards the firming up of vocabulary skills (Sowell et al., 2004) in relationship with improvements in phonological skills (Lu et al., 2007). Consequently, analysts are teasing aside the brain-based distinctions which may be noticed before children begin to work out how to read from variations that may occur because of less reading by individuals who have dyslexia. For example, experts have found modified brain anatomy (Raschle, et al., 2011) and function (Raschle, et al., 2012) in pre-reading children with a family group background of dyslexia. Future studies using longitudinal designs (i.e., long-term), will inform the timeline from the adjustments and clarify cause and ramifications of anatomical and practical distinctions in dyslexia.

CHAPTER 8

Overview of Intervention found in Brain imaging research of Children with RD

The average person tutoring intervention occurred day-by-day for fifty minutes from September to June, which yielded typically 100 and twenty-six sessions or 100 and five tutoring hours per student.

Instruction

Each session contains a framework of five steps that tutors followed with each student. This platform had not been scripted but was individualized predicated on the student's improvement.

1.   Short and quick-paced summary of sound-symbol human relationships from previous lessons and intro of new correspondences.

2.   Term work practice of phonemic segmentation and mixing with letter charge cards or tiles, which occurred

in an extremely systematic and explicit fashion.

3.   Fluency building with view of words and phonetically regular words composed of previously taught sound-symbol correspondences.

4.   Dental reading practice in phonetically managed text, uncontrolled trade books, and non-fiction texts.

5.   Writing words with previously taught patterns from dictation.

The intervention contains six levels that started with simple closed syllable words (e.g., kitty) and finished with multisyllabic words comprising all six syllable types.

Prior to the intervention, all groups looked similar of their brain activity, but soon after the intervention, the experimental and control groups had increased activation in the quit hemispheric region very crucial that you read.

A year after intervention, the experimental group showed increased activity in the occipito-temporal region very crucial that you automated, fluent reading, while at both time factors the amount of compensatory activation in the correct hemisphere decreased.

Shaywitz et al. (2002) concluded, "These results indicate that the usage of the evidence-based phonologic reading treatment facilitates the development of the fast-paced neural systems that underlie skilled reading".

Important considerations to notice about your brain research.

While research advances have allowed us to look more closely within your brain for the very first time and revealed important info about how precisely and might know about thinking while reading, there are necessary considerations that basically should be remembered.

You are that as well as the report by B.E. Shaywitz, S. Shaywitz, and their co-workers, the test sizes in each research are actually small. The knowledge from these small studies is converging into results that are reliable, however the results may change as far more folks are within the study foundation. This is also true with children where both degree of studies as well as the test sizes have grown to be small.

Second, we must consider the sort of job being inside the magnet. Due to the need the individuals brain won't undertake the imaging, researchers cannot research people actually reading aloud. Instead, they provide tasks trying the individual to learn silently and decide that he/she shows using a drive button (e.g., Do the characters - t and v rhyme? Do leat and jete rhyme?).

As professionals have been employed carefully on these tasks and possess also specified this system that's measured, we're able to trust their conclusions in what the activation amounts mean; however, the jobs have become removed natural class reading and could not be interpreted as though these were the same. The location of brain research is developing quickly; technological improvements are being made that may address these issues later on.

Options for Teachers

What does all this info mean for college staff and their students? Once educators realise the primary processes and factors behind reading disabilities, they might use this info because they connect to students and themselves. Listed below are specific suggestions predicated in the neurological research:

· Sufficient assessment of language processing is important in identifying why students battle to regulate how exactly to learn.

· Dyslexia, or reading impairment, can be a problem of the vocabulary control systems in your brain. Specific information regarding precisely what types of weaknesses can be found must be capable of looking for the right teaching to meet each student's needs.

· Imaging research confirms that easy jobs could possibly be a lot more reliably interpreted as "warning flag" suggesting a kid could be in peril for dyslexia.

· It is key to begin using testing and improvement monitoring procedures in first stages to measure children's knowledge of sound in speech, notice sound in words, and fluent term reputation. Using such evaluation within an ongoing way within a child's college profession will help instructors know very well what skills to instruct and whether a young child is normally developing these skills.

Explicit, intense, systematic instructions in the audio structure of vocabulary (phonemic recognition) and in how sound connect with words (phonics) is vital for people who have dyslexia.

Imaging research verified that instruction in the alphabetic principle triggered distinct variations in brain activation patterns in the students with RD (Shaywitz et al., 2004). Understand that the task was explicit, extreme, long-term, and specifically centred on phonological handling, phonics, and fluency.

The roles of motivation and nervous about failing are necessary when discussing reading problems.

Students will not struggle simply because they aren't trying hard enough. They could have a brain difference that may require these to understand within a lot more extreme way than their peers. Without extreme intervention, low inspiration may develop as students avoid a hard and painful task.

School personnel might use their understanding of the neurological characteristics and basis of dyslexia to help their students understand their advantages and weaknesses around reading and vocabulary.

Understanding a possible reason, they could learn something difficult that nobody else appears to struggle with that will assist relieve a number of the mystery and negative feelings a lot of individuals who've a disability encounter. Sharing our understanding of brain research would demystify dyslexia, and help students and their parents observe that vocabulary processing is just about the many talents they have and they also aren't "ridiculous"; they simply process vocabulary in various ways than their peers.

CHAPTER 9

Practical Brain Differences

One common way for imaging brain function is Functional Magnetic Resonance Imaging (fMRI), a noninvasive, relatively new technique that actions physiological indicators of neural activation employing a strong magnet to pinpoint blood flow. This method is known as "practical" because individuals perform jobs while in (or under) the magnet, allowing dimension from the working brain instead of the experience of the mind at rest.

Many studies using useful imaging techniques that compared the mind activation patterns of readers with and without dyslexia show potentially crucial patterns of differences. We might expect that folks with RD would display under-activation in areas where they might be weaker and over-activation in the areas, which is usually just what many experts have found (e.g., Shaywitz et al., 1998).

This type of functional imaging research has just been utilized with children. That's partly due to the down sides associated with imaging children, just like the absolute reliance on the participant's have a look at to stay motionless through the scanning.

We will present the largest, best-specified study for instance of the brand new results with children. Shaywitz et al. (2002) researched a hundred and forty-four ideal handed children with and without RD on several in- and out-of-magnet responsibilities; the likened brain activation in the middle of your two sets of children on jobs made to faucet several component procedures of reading are:

· identifying the titles or seems of letters.

· sounding out nonsense words.

· sounding out and evaluating meanings of real words.

The non-impaired readers had even more activation from the areas regarded to as very vital compared to the kids with dyslexia.

Shaywitz et al. (2002) also found that the children who've been sound decoders experienced even more activation in the areas very vital that reading in the quit hemisphere and less in the proper hemisphere compared to the kids with RD.

They suggested that for children with RD, disruption in the trunk reading systems in the left hemisphere that are necessary for skilled, fluent reading, leads the youngsters to compensate through the use of other, less efficient systems.

This finding could clarify the standard experience in school that whilst children with dyslexia become accurate readers, their reading in grade-level text is often still slow and laboured without fluency (e.g., Torgesen, Rashotte, & Alexander, 2001).

In summary, the mind of the individual with dyslexia includes a different distribution of metabolic activation compared to the brain of the individual without reading problems when accomplishing the same vocabulary task. There are failing from the left hemisphere back brain systems to use properly during reading.

Furthermore, many individuals who have dyslexia often show greater activation in the reduced frontal parts of the mind. This leads to the ultimate result that neural systems in frontal areas may compensate for the disruption in the posterior area (Shaywitz et al., 2003). This info often lead teachers to question whether brain imaging can be employed like a diagnostic tool to identify children with reading disabilities in college.

Can we display everyone which has reading difficulties?

Not yet. It truly is an attractive eyesight of putting a youngster we come to mind about in a fMRI machine to quickly and accurately identify his/her problem, but research hasn't used it very much.

There are numerous explanations to why a clinical or school-based usage of imaging methods to identify children with dyslexia isn't presently feasible. The foremost is the tremendous cost of fMRI machines, the personal computers, and this program had a need to run them. Another section of the cost may be the personnel that's needed is to perform and interpret the results.

Also, because of this technology to be used for diagnosis, it needs to become accurate for folks. Currently, email details are reliable and reported for sets of participants; however, definitely not for folks within each group (Richards, 2001; Shaywitz et al., 2002).

The quantity of children who are identified to become average if they obviously have a problem (false negatives), or as utilizing a problem when they are average (false positives) would need to be significantly lower for imaging methods to be used for diagnosis of individual children.

Acknowledgements

The Glory of this book success goes to God Almighty and my beautiful Family, Fans, Readers & well-wishers, Customers, and Friends for their endless support and encouragement.